THE ANTI-INFLAMMATORY DIET SLOW COOKER COOKBOOK

"Simple and Delicious Slow Cooker Recipes for a Healthier, Anti-Inflammatory Lifestyle"

By

GINA .P. ERIN

Copyright © 2024 by Gina P. Erin

Copyright is fully asserted. Unauthorized replication, dissemination, or broadcasting of any segment of this publication, through photocopying, audio recording, or via electronic or mechanical techniques, is strictly forbidden without the publisher's formal consent in writing. This excludes short excerpts used in scholarly critiques and specific non-profit activities sanctioned by copyright law.

DISCLAIMER

This book is meant solely for informational and educational enhancement and shouldn't be seen as medical counsel. The author isn't a health expert, and this book's content shouldn't replace professional medical guidance, diagnosis, or care. Always consult with your doctor or a qualified health professional for any health-related questions.

The author won't be held accountable for any direct or indirect outcomes from using this book. The material is presented "as is" without any guarantees, either clear or implied. The author does not guarantee the accuracy or fullness of this book's contents and expressly renounces any warranties of saleability or suitability for any specific use.

The recipes are for informational aims only. The author is not responsible for any negative reactions or other consequences from using or misapplying these recipes.

Trademarks and registered trademarks found in this book belong to their respective holders. Their appearance does not imply any endorsement or connection.

TABLE OF CONTENT

ABOUT THE AUTHOR

INTRODUCTION

CHAPTER 1: BREAKFAST

Recipe 1. Sweet Potato Home Fries

Recipe 2. Caramel- apple oat

Recipe 3. Perfect Hard-boiled egg

Recipe 4: Carrot and Fennel Quinoa

Recipe 5:. Chicken -Apple Breakfast Sausage

Recipe 6: Breakfast Casserole

Recipe 7: Sour Cherry and Pumpkin Seed Granola

Recipe 8: Morning Millet

Recipe 9: Protein Oat

Recipe 10: German Chocolate cake

CHAPTER 2: Sauces and Staples

Recipe 1: Vanilla-Pear butter

Recipe 2: Vegan Buffalo Dip

Recipe 3: Chimichurri Sauce

Recipe 4: Creamy Tumeric dressing

Recipe 5: Strawberry and Chia Seed Jam

Recipe 6: Caramelized onions

Recipe 7: Tangy Barbecue sauce with Apple Cider vinegar

Recipe 8: Old-fashioned Applesauce

Recipe 9: Avocado-Dill Sauce

Recipe 10: Garden Marinara sauce

CHAPTER 3: Plant-Based Mains

Recipe 1: White Beans and French Onions Soup

Recipe 2: Masala Lentil

Recipe 3: Minestrone Soup
Recipe 4: Jam-packed Pepper
Recipe 5: Wild rice Soup with Mushrooms
Recipe 6: Balsamic Beet
Recipe 7: Indian-Spice Cauliflower
Recipe 8: Golden Lentil Soup
Recipe 9: Classic Vegetable Broth
Recipe 10: Stuffed Sweet Potatoes
Review

ABOUT THE AUTHOR

Meet Gina P. Erin, a culinary whiz whose heart beats for the healthy food movement. With a seasoned background in the kitchen and a deep-seated passion for nutrition, Gina stands out in the foodie universe for whipping up scrumptious, health-centric dishes that do more than just please the palate—they enrich your well-being.

Gina's voyage into the realm of wholesome noshing took off from her early days in the culinary trenches. Fueled by curiosity about food's influence on health, she's dedicated hours on end to playing with ingredients and refining her cooking methods. The result? Recipes that pack a punch in both taste and nutrients. She's got a soft spot for natural, unadulterated foods that are kind to your body. Home is where the heart is, and for Gina, it's also where she concocts her culinary magic.

A happily married chef, she finds joy and inspiration in the rhythms of her home life and her professional escapades. For Gina, food is more than sustenance—it's a catalyst for camaraderie and wellness.

Her philosophy extends beyond the plate; it's about curating moments that elevate life's flavor. Through her cookbooks, Gina spills the beans on her wholesome eating ethos, dishing out savvy advice, detailed nutrition facts, and a smorgasbord of mouthwatering recipes.

Her recent creation, ' THE ANTI- INFLAMMATORY DIET SLOW COOKER COOKBOOK' is a nod to her dedication to making wholesome chow fun and accessible to all. Embark on a gastronomic adventure with Gina P. Erin and savor the blend of culinary artistry and nutritional wisdom. It's a journey that promises to reshape your relationship with food and lead you to a more mindful, healthful existence.

INTRODUCTION

The Slow Cooker Cookbook: Anti-Inflammatory Diet
Millions of individuals worldwide are impacted by the hidden pandemic of chronic inflammation that has emerged in a world of processed foods and fast-paced life. Although persistent inflammation is the body's normal reaction to damage or sickness, it may also cause a number of other health issues, such as diabetes, heart disease, arthritis, and even certain types of cancer. The good news is that our diets may significantly affect our body's inflammatory levels.

The Anti-Inflammatory Diet is a way of life that prioritizes full, nutrient-dense foods that support general health, heal the body, and reduce inflammation. It's not simply a diet.

For those who want to enjoy healthful, anti-inflammatory meals without spending hours in the kitchen, the slow cooker—a cherished household appliance renowned for its simplicity and convenience—offers the ideal option. This cookbook makes it simpler than ever to establish good eating habits that may drastically improve your health by fusing the anti-inflammatory diet's tenets with the ease of slow cooking.

With an emphasis on foods that lower inflammation, this cookbook offers a broad range of dishes to suit all palates and dietary requirements. These recipes, which range from filling soups and stews to delicate meats and colorful vegetable dishes, are designed to maximize taste and nutrition with the least amount of work. Scientific research has shown that anti-inflammatory nutrients including leafy greens, colorful vegetables, fatty fish, nuts, seeds, and spices like ginger and turmeric may help decrease inflammation and promote general health. These ingredients are carefully chosen to incorporate anti-inflammatory elements in each dish.

This cookbook is an excellent resource for learning how to eat in a manner that feeds your body and reduces inflammation, regardless of your goals—be they weight loss, improved energy levels, or managing a particular health problem. Simple recipes and readily available components allow you to make delicious, therapeutic meals that help you achieve your health objectives.

With the help of the Anti-Inflammatory Diet Slow Cooker Cookbook, embrace the path to improved health. Let's start cooking to move toward a life free of inflammation and well-being.

In a world filled with fast-paced living and processed foods, chronic inflammation has become a silent epidemic affecting millions of people. Inflammation is the body's natural response to injury or illness, but when it becomes chronic, it can lead to a host of health problems, including heart disease, diabetes, arthritis, and even certain cancers. The good news is that what we eat can have a significant impact on inflammation levels in the body. The Anti-Inflammatory Diet is not just a diet; it's a lifestyle that emphasizes whole, nutrient-dense foods that fight inflammation, heal the body, and promote overall well-being.

The slow cooker, a beloved kitchen tool known for its convenience and ease, provides the perfect solution for those who want to enjoy wholesome, anti-inflammatory meals without spending hours in the kitchen. This cookbook brings together the principles of the anti-inflammatory diet with the simplicity of slow cooking, making it easier than ever to adopt healthy eating habits that can transform your health.

In this cookbook, you'll find a wide array of recipes that cater to different tastes and dietary preferences, all while focusing on foods that reduce inflammation. From hearty soups and stews to tender meats and vibrant vegetable dishes, these recipes are crafted to provide maximum flavor and nutrition with minimal effort. Each recipe is carefully designed to include anti-inflammatory ingredients such as leafy greens, colorful vegetables, fatty fish, nuts, seeds, and spices like turmeric and ginger—all of which have been scientifically proven to help reduce inflammation and support overall health.

Whether you're looking to manage a specific health condition, lose weight, or simply feel better and more energized, this cookbook is your guide to eating in a way that nourishes your body and calms inflammation. With easy-to-follow instructions and accessible ingredients, you can create delicious, healing meals that support your health goals.

Embrace the journey to better health with the Anti-Inflammatory Diet Slow Cooker Cookbook. Let's get cooking and take the first step towards a healthier, inflammation-free life!

CHAPTER 1: BREAKFAST

The Most Important Meal of the Day is Breakfast

There's good reason why breakfast is often referred to as the most significant meal of the day. It breaks the time of fasting throughout the night, replaces your glucose reserves to increase alertness and energy, and gives you the vital nutrients needed for good health. A well-balanced breakfast may help you stay energized, focused, and prepared to take on the day's challenges.

Recipe 1: Sweet Potato Home Fries

Servings: 4
Prep Time: 10 minutes
Cook Time: 25 minutes

Ingredients:

2 large sweet potatoes, peeled and diced into 1/2-inch cubes (about 4 cups)
1 medium red onion, diced
1 red bell pepper, diced
2 tablespoons olive oil
1 teaspoon garlic powder
1 teaspoon smoked paprika
1/2 teaspoon ground cumin
Salt and black pepper, to taste
2 tablespoons fresh parsley, chopped (optional, for garnish)

Nutritional Facts (Per Serving):

Calories: 180

Protein: 2g

Carbohydrates: 30g

Dietary Fiber: 5g

Total Sugars: 7g

Total Fat: 7g

Saturated Fat: 1g

Preparation

1. Turn up the heat to high and get ready: Preheat your slow cooker. Peel the sweet potatoes and chop them into consistent 1/2-inch cubes for even cooking while the oven preheats. Chop the red onion and red bell pepper into pieces of a comparable size.

2. Ingredients: Combine the sweet potatoes, chopped onion, and bell pepper in a big bowl and toss to coat thoroughly with the olive oil, smoked paprika, ground cumin, garlic powder, and black pepper.

3. Use the Slow Cooker to Cook: Place the seasoned sweet potato mixture in the slow cooker that has been prepared. Sweet potatoes should be cooked for two to three hours on high,

covered, and with slightly crisped edges. Cook the fries for a little longer if you'd like them softer.

4. Complete and Serve: After cooking, taste for seasoning and add more salt or pepper if necessary. If preferred, garnish with freshly cut parsley for extra taste and a splash of color. Enjoy as a nutritious snack or heated as a side dish.

This meal is a great complement to an anti-inflammatory diet since it's tasty, simple to make, and full of vitamins and fiber. Please let me know if you want any further information or recipes!

Recipe 2. Caramel- apple oat

Servings: 4
Prep Time: 10 minutes
Cook Time: 6-8 hours (slow cooker setting on low)

Ingredients:
1 1/2 cups steel-cut oats
4 cups unsweetened almond milk (or milk of choice)
2 medium apples, peeled, cored, and diced
1/4 cup pure maple syrup
1 tablespoon unsweetened applesauce

1 teaspoon ground cinnamon

1/2 teaspoon ground nutmeg

1 teaspoon vanilla extract

1/4 teaspoon salt

2 tablespoons unsalted butter or coconut oil

1/4 cup chopped pecans (optional, for topping)

2 tablespoons caramel sauce (optional, for drizzling)

Nutritional Facts (Per Serving):

Calories: 320

Protein: 7g

Carbohydrates: 56g

Dietary Fiber: 7g

Total Sugars: 20g

Total Fat: 9g

Saturated Fat: 3g

Preparation

1.Set Up the Slow Cooker: To keep the oats from sticking, lightly coat the inside of a slow cooker with coconut oil or unsalted butter.

2.Combine Ingredients: Fill the slow cooker with the steel-cut oats, unsweetened almond milk, chopped apples, maple syrup, applesauce, ground nutmeg, ground cinnamon, vanilla essence, and salt. To uniformly mix all the ingredients, give it a good stir.

3.simmer on Low: Preheat the slow cooker to low and simmer the oats and apples for 6 to 8 hours, or overnight, until the oats are creamy and tender.

4.Add Butter and Serve: For a rich, caramel-like taste, mix in 2 tablespoons unsalted butter or coconut oil just before serving. If preferred, garnish with chopped pecans and a thin layer of caramel sauce and serve hot.

5.Optional Toppings: For extra nourishment, top your caramel apple oatmeal with chopped bananas, raisins, or a sprinkling of flax seeds.

Packed with protein, fiber, and other vital minerals, this Caramel Apple Oatmeal is a wonderful blend of sweet and savory tastes. It's a simple and satisfying meal that is good for reducing inflammation.

Recipe 3. Perfect Hard-boiled egg

Servings: 4
Prep Time: 5 minutes
Cook Time: 10-12 minutes
Total Time: 17 minutes

Ingredients:
8 large eggs
Water (enough to cover the eggs by 1 inch)
Ice (for an ice bath)

Nutritional Facts (Per Egg):
Calories: 70
Protein: 6g
Carbohydrates: 0g
Dietary Fiber: 0g
Total Sugars: 0g
Total Fat: 5g
Saturated Fat: 1.5g

Preparation:
1. Egg preparation: Fill a medium saucepan with eggs, arranging them in a single layer at the bottom. Pour in enough cold water to come up to approximately an inch over the eggs.

Bring the water to a rolling boil by placing the saucepan over medium-high heat.

2. Cook the Eggs: Place a lid on the pot and turn off the heat as soon as the water reaches a roaring boil. Depending on the consistency you want for the yolks, let the eggs in the boiling water for 10 to 12 minutes.

3. For ten minutes: middle of yolk somewhat creamy.
12 minutes: The yolk is hard and fully set.
As the eggs are frying, prepare an ice bath by filling a big dish with ice water.

4. Cool the Eggs: Using a slotted spoon, quickly move the cooked eggs to the ice bath. Give them at least five minutes to sit in the icy water. This halts the heating process and facilitates peeling.

5. Peel and Serve: Crack the eggshells gently by tapping each one on a hard surface. Then, peel them under cold running water. The hard-boiled eggs may be served right away or kept for up to a week in the refrigerator.

6. Perfect Hard-Boiled Eggs are a nutrient-dense, adaptable snack or side dish for any dinner. They are a fantastic addition to any anti-inflammatory diet since they are a terrific source of critical vitamins, healthy fats, and high-quality protein.

Recipe 4: Carrot and Fennel Quinoa

Servings: 4
Prep Time: 10 minutes
Cook Time: 20 minutes
Total Time: 30 minutes

Ingredients:
1 cup quinoa, rinsed and drained
2 cups vegetable broth or water
1 medium fennel bulb, trimmed, cored, and thinly sliced
2 medium carrots, peeled and shredded

1 tablespoon olive oil
2 cloves garlic, minced
1/2 teaspoon ground cumin
1/2 teaspoon ground coriander
Salt and black pepper, to taste
2 tablespoons fresh parsley, chopped
1 tablespoon lemon juice
1/4 cup feta cheese, crumbled (optional)

Nutritional Facts (Per Serving):
Calories: 210
Protein: 6g

Carbohydrates: 32g
Dietary Fiber: 5g
Total Sugars: 5g
Total Fat: 6g
Saturated Fat: 1g

1. Cook the Quinoa: Bring water or vegetable broth to a boil in a medium saucepan. When the quinoa is cooked and all of the liquid has been absorbed, around 15 minutes should pass after adding the rinsed quinoa, lowering the heat to low, covering, and simmering. Using a fork, fluff and put aside.

2. Sauté the Vegetables: In a large pan set over medium heat, heat the olive oil while the quinoa cooks. Add the sliced fennel and simmer, stirring periodically, until the fennel starts to soften, approximately 5 minutes.

3. Add the ground cumin, ground coriander, minced garlic, and shredded carrots to the pan along with the spices. Put some salt and black pepper over it. Stirring often, cook the veggies for a further five minutes or until they are soft and aromatic.

4. Quinoa and veggies Together: Put the cooked quinoa and the sautéed veggies in a pan. Toss to thoroughly mix in all the

ingredients. Cook for two more minutes to ensure it is well heated.

To finish and serve, take off the heat source and mix in the lemon juice and fresh parsley. If necessary, taste and adjust the seasoning. If preferred, garnish the heated dish with crumbled feta cheese.

5. Fennel with Carrots An anti-inflammatory diet would benefit greatly from the nutrient-dense, tasty, and light quinoa meal. This meal is a tasty and nutritious choice for lunch or supper since it is strong in fiber, vitamins, and minerals.

Recipe 5:.Chicken -Apple Breakfast Sausage

Servings: 6 (makes about 12 patties)
Prep Time: 15 minutes
Cook Time: 10 minutes
Total Time: 25 minutes

Ingredients:
-1 pound ground chicken (preferably lean)
-1 medium apple (Granny Smith or Honeycrisp), peeled, cored, and grated
-1/4 cup onion, finely diced
-2 cloves garlic, minced
-1 tablespoon fresh sage, finely chopped (or 1 teaspoon dried sage)

-1 teaspoon fresh thyme, finely chopped (or 1/2 teaspoon dried thyme)
-1/2 teaspoon ground cinnamon
-1/4 teaspoon ground nutmeg
-1/4 teaspoon ground black pepper
-1/2 teaspoon salt
-1 tablespoon olive oil or avocado oil (for cooking)

Nutritional Facts (Per Serving - 2 Patties):
Calories: 140
Protein: 18g
Carbohydrates: 4g
Dietary Fiber: 0.5g
Total Sugars: 2g
Total Fat: 6g
Saturated Fat: 1g

Preparation
1. Preparing the Mixture: Put the ground chicken, grated apple, sliced onion, minced garlic, cinnamon, nutmeg, black pepper, and salt in a big bowl. Until all of the ingredients are combined evenly, stir. Avoid overmixing as this might result in tough sausages.

2. Shape the Patties: Using your hands, shape the mixture into 12 little patties, each with a diameter of around 2 inches. To

guarantee consistent cooking, make sure they are of the same size.

3.Prepare the Sausages: In a big skillet, warm the olive oil over medium heat. When heated through, place the patties in a single layer (batch cooking may be necessary). Cook for about 4–5 minutes on each side, or until they are cooked through and have an internal temperature of 165°F (74°C), becoming golden brown.

4.To serve, take out of the pan and drain on a platter covered with paper towels to get rid of any extra oil. Serve warm with eggs, avocado, or sautéed veggies for a hearty breakfast.

5.Storage Advice: You can freeze these sausages for up to two months or keep them in the refrigerator for up to three days when kept in an airtight container. Place them in a pan over medium heat and reheat until well hot.

6.Chicken-Apple Breakfast Sausage, with the sweetness of apples and the savory flavors of herbs and spices, provides a tasty, high-protein start to your day. This dish is a better option for an anti-inflammatory diet since it doesn't include any preservatives as store-bought alternatives do.

Recipe 6: Breakfast Casserole

Servings: 8 per serving
Prep Time: 15 minutes
Cook Time: 40 minutes
Total Time: 55 minutes

Ingredients:
- 8 large eggs
- 1 cup milk (dairy or non-dairy)
- 1/2 cup shredded cheddar cheese (or dairy-free alternative)
- 1/2 cup shredded mozzarella cheese (or dairy-free alternative)
- 1/2 pound ground turkey or chicken sausage (or plant-based sausage)
- 1 medium onion, diced
- 1 bell pepper, diced (red, yellow, or green)
- 2 cups baby spinach, chopped
- 2 cups frozen hash browns, thawed
- 1/2 teaspoon garlic powder
- 1/2 teaspoon paprika
- Salt and black pepper, to taste
- 1 tablespoon olive oil

Nutritional Facts (Per Serving):
- Calories: 220
- Protein: 14g
- Carbohydrates: 10g
- Dietary Fiber: 1g
- Total Sugars: 2g
- Total Fat: 14g
- Saturated Fat: 4g

Preparation:

1. Preheat the Oven: Set the oven's temperature to 375°F, or 190°C. Spray cooking spray or lightly coat a 9 x 13-inch baking dish with olive oil.

2. Prepare the veggies and sausage: One tablespoon of olive oil should be heated in a big pan over medium heat. Add the ground turkey or chicken sausage and heat for 5 to 7 minutes, or until browned and thoroughly cooked. After taking the sausage out of the pan, put it aside. Add the diced onion and bell pepper to the same skillet. Sauté until softened, 3–4 minutes. Cook the chopped spinach for a further one to two minutes, or until it wilts.

3. Get the Egg Mixture Ready: Mix the eggs, milk, paprika, garlic powder, salt, and black pepper in a big bowl. Add the mozzarella and cheddar cheeses that have been shredded.

4. Put the Casserole Together: Fill the baking dish with the thawed hash browns equally. Arrange the hash browns in a layer with the cooked sausage and the sautéed veggies. Making sure that every ingredient is coated equally, pour the egg mixture over the top.

5. Prepare the casserole by baking: Bake for 35 to 40 minutes, or until the top is golden brown and the eggs are set, in a preheated oven. A toothpick or knife inserted in the middle should come out clean when the food is done.

6. Assist: Before slicing, let the casserole cool for about five minutes. Garnish with more cheese or fresh herbs and serve warm.

7. Storage Advice: You may keep leftover casserole in the fridge for up to three days if you put it in an airtight container. Warm up individual servings in the oven or microwave until well heated.

This filling, high-protein breakfast casserole canis ideal for meal prep or serving a large audience. Rich in tasty cheeses, lean protein, and wholesome veggies, it's a great choice for a diet that reduces inflammation. Tell me if you need any more recipes or modifications!

Recipe 7: Sour Cherry and Pumpkin Seed Granola

Servings: 8 (1/2 cup per serving)

Prep Time: 10 minutes
Cook Time: 30 minutes
Total Time: 40 minutes

Ingredients:
3 cups old-fashioned rolled oats
1 cup raw pumpkin seeds
1/2 cup unsweetened shredded coconut
1/2 cup raw almonds, chopped
1/4 cup chia seeds
1/4 cup flaxseeds
1/2 cup dried sour cherries, roughly chopped
1/3 cup honey or maple syrup
1/4 cup coconut oil, melted
1 teaspoon vanilla extract
1 teaspoon ground cinnamon
1/4 teaspoon salt

Nutritional Facts (Per Serving):

Calories: 290

Protein: 8g

Carbohydrates: 35g

Dietary Fiber: 6g

Total Sugars: 12g

Total Fat: 14g

Saturated Fat: 6g

Preparation:

1. Set the Oven's Temperature to 325°F (163°C). Put parchment paper on the bottom of a large baking sheet.

2. Combine the dry ingredients in a big bowl: add the rolled oats, ground cinnamon, chia seeds, flaxseeds, sliced almonds, pumpkin seeds, and shredded coconut. For all components to be distributed evenly, thoroughly mix.

3. To prepare the wet ingredients, mix the melted coconut oil, vanilla extract, and honey or maple syrup in a small bowl and whisk until well incorporated.

Integrate the dry and wet ingredients: Over the dry mixture, pour the wet ingredients. Using a wooden spoon or spatula, thoroughly stir the dry ingredients until they are completely covered.

4.Spread and Bake: Evenly spread the granola mixture onto the baking sheet that has been ready. Bake for 25 to 30 minutes in a preheated oven, stirring every 10 minutes to achieve uniform baking and avoid scorching. The granola should smell aromatic and become a golden brown.

5.Add Dried Cherries: Take the granola out of the oven and allow it to cool fully on the baking sheet when it has finished baking. Stir in the chopped dry sour cherries when it has cooled. As it cools, the granola will become crispy.

6.Store and Serve: After the granola cools down, move it to an airtight jar and keep it chilled for up to two weeks. Savor it by itself, as a topping for yogurt, or as a filling breakfast alternative with milk.

A tasty and high-nutrient granola dish, Sour Cherry and Pumpkin Seed Granola mixes the crunch of almonds and pumpkin seeds with the sharpness of dried cherries. Rich in protein, healthy fats, and fiber, it's a fantastic anti-inflammatory breakfast or snack.

Recipe 8: Morning Millet

Servings: 4
Prep Time: 5 minutes
Cook Time: 25 minutes
Total Time: 30 minutes

Ingredients:
- 1 cup millet, rinsed and drained
- 2 cups water or unsweetened almond milk (or any milk of choice)
- 1/2 teaspoon ground cinnamon
- 1/4 teaspoon ground nutmeg
- 1/4 teaspoon salt
- 1 tablespoon maple syrup or honey (optional)
- 1/4 cup chopped nuts (almonds, walnuts, or pecans)
- 1/4 cup dried fruits (raisins, cranberries, or chopped dates)
- 1 medium apple or pear, diced
- 1 tablespoon chia seeds or flaxseeds (optional)

Nutritional Facts (Per Serving):
- Calories: 230
- Protein: 6g
- Carbohydrates: 42g
- Dietary Fiber: 5g
- Total Sugars: 9g
- Total Fat: 6g
- Saturated Fat: 1g

Preparation:

1. Toasted Millet: Place the rinsed and drained millet in a medium saucepan and place over medium heat. Stirring frequently, toast the millet for 3–4 minutes until aromatic and beginning to become golden. This process brings out the millet's nutty taste.

2. Cook the Millet: Put the toasted millet in a pot and add two cups of water or unsweetened almond milk. Add the salt, ground nutmeg, and cinnamon and stir. After bringing the mixture to a boil, turn down the heat. For fifteen to twenty minutes, or until the millet is soft and the liquid has been absorbed, cover the pot and simmer.

3. Add Sweetener and Toppings: Take the pot off of the burner and, if you're using it, whisk in the honey or maple syrup. Add the chopped nuts, dried fruits, and diced apple or pear and fold gently. Add some flaxseeds or chia seeds for an added nutritious boost.

4. To serve, portion out the millet into bowls and reheat them up. If preferred, sprinkle some more almonds, dried fruit, or maple syrup on top.

5. Storage Advice: You may keep leftover millet in the fridge for up to three days if you keep it in an airtight container. To loosen the texture, reheat in the microwave or on the stovetop while adding a splash of milk or water.

A filling and wholesome breakfast alternative, morning millet is high in fiber, protein, and vital vitamins and minerals. As a fantastic gluten-free substitute for typical grains, millet is perfect for an anti-inflammatory diet. Please inquire if you want any more recipes or modifications!

Recipe 9: Protein Oat

Servings: 2
Prep Time: 5 minutes
Cook Time: 5 minutes
Total Time: 10 minutes

Ingredients:
1 cup old-fashioned rolled oats
1 1/2 cups unsweetened almond milk (or any milk of choice)
1 scoop (about 30g) vanilla protein powder (whey, pea, or your choice)
1 tablespoon chia seeds or flaxseeds
1 tablespoon almond butter or peanut butter
1/2 teaspoon ground cinnamon
1/4 teaspoon salt

1/4 cup fresh berries (strawberries, blueberries, or raspberries)
1 tablespoon honey or maple syrup (optional)
2 tablespoons chopped nuts (almonds, walnuts, or pecans)

Nutritional Facts (Per Serving):
Calories: 320
Protein: 20g
Carbohydrates: 38g

Dietary Fiber: 8g
Total Sugars: 8g
Total Fat: 10g
Saturated Fat: 1g

Preparation

1. Cook the Oats: Place the rolled oats and unsweetened almond milk in a medium pot and heat. After bringing to a low simmer, cook, stirring regularly, for three to five minutes, or until the mixture has thickened and the oats are soft.

2. After the oats are cooked, take the pot from the stove and add the protein powder. Add the almond butter, ground cinnamon, protein powder, chia or flaxseeds, and salt.

3.Stir well to ensure that all the ingredients are properly combined. The consistency of the oats should be creamy. To get the right texture, thin down any excess mixture by adding a little amount of more milk.

4.Sweeten and Serve: If you'd like your oats sweeter, taste them and add honey or maple syrup. Split the protein-rich oats into two separate bowls.

5.Place a top and savor: For extra taste and texture, sprinkle chopped nuts and fresh berries over the top of each dish. While still heated, serve right away.

6.Storage Advice: You may keep leftover protein oats in the fridge for up to three days if you keep them in an airtight container.

7.Warm up in the microwave or on the stovetop while stirring and adding a splash of milk until well heated.

A great high-protein, high-fiber breakfast choice that will keep you satisfied and energetic all morning long are protein oats. This recipe's healthful fats from nuts and seeds, together with the protein powder and oats, making it perfect for an anti-inflammatory diet.

Recipe 10: German Chocolate cake

Servings: 12
Prep Time: 30 minutes
Cook Time: 30 minutes
Total Time: 1 hour + cooling time

Ingredients:
For the Cake:
1/2 cup unsweetened cocoa powder
1/2 cup boiling water
1 cup buttermilk, room temperature
1 teaspoon vanilla extract
2 cups all-purpose flour
1 1/2 teaspoons baking soda
1/2 teaspoon baking powder
1/2 teaspoon salt
1 cup unsalted butter, softened
1 1/2 cups granulated sugar
1/2 cup packed light brown sugar
4 large eggs, room temperature

For the Coconut-Pecan Frosting:
1 cup evaporated milk
1 cup granulated sugar
3 large egg yolks, beaten
1/2 cup unsalted butter, cut into pieces

1 teaspoon vanilla extract
1 1/2 cups sweetened shredded coconut
1 cup chopped pecans

Nutritional Facts (Per Serving):
Calories: 570
Protein: 7g
Carbohydrates: 68g
Dietary Fiber: 3g
Total Sugars: 47g
Total Fat: 31g
Saturated Fat: 17g

Preparation
1. Set the oven temperature to 350°F (175°C). Three 9-inch round cake pans should be floured, greased, and have parchment paper placed within the bottoms.
2. Boil the water and the unsweetened cocoa powder in a small dish. Once smooth, stir and set aside to cool.

3. Whisk the vanilla essence and buttermilk together in a separate dish and put it aside.
Sift flour, baking powder, baking soda, and salt in a medium-sized basin; put aside.

4. Blend the Cake Ingredients:

Using an electric mixer set to medium speed, beat the butter, brown sugar, and granulated sugar in a large mixing basin until light and fluffy, approximately 3 minutes.

5. One egg at a time, add them, beating well after each addition.

6. Beginning and finishing with the flour combination, alternately add the buttermilk mixture and flour mixture to the butter mixture. Beat only till everything is included. Add the chilled cocoa mixture and stir.

7. Cook the Layers of Cake: Using three prepared pans, divide the batter equally. Use a spatula to smooth the tops. If a toothpick is pushed into the middle, it should come out clean after 25 to 30 minutes of baking in a preheated oven.

8. After allowing the cakes to cool in the pans for ten minutes, take them out and place them on wire racks to finish cooling.

9. Get the Pecan-Coconut Frosting ready: Combine the butter, egg yolks, sugar, and evaporated milk in a medium saucepan over medium heat. Cook for approximately 12 minutes, stirring continuously, or until the liquid thickens and becomes golden brown.

Take off the heat and mix in the chopped pecans, shredded coconut, and vanilla extract. The frosting will thicken as it cools, so let it reach room temperature.

Put the Cake Together: Arrange a single layer of cake onto a platter. Evenly cover the top with a third of the coconut-pecan icing. Top with the second layer, then cover with an additional third of the frosting. Spread the remaining frosting over the top of the cake after placing the last layer on top.

Serve: Cake should be served room temperature after slicing. Any leftovers may be kept in the fridge for up to five days if they are kept in an airtight container. Before serving, bring to room temperature.

German Chocolate Cake is a rich and luscious delicacy distinguished by its distinct coconut-pecan icing and creamy chocolate layers. This traditional cake is ideal for get-togethers and special events.

CHAPTER 3: Sauces and Staples

Recipe 1: Vanilla-Pear butter

Servings: 24 (1 tablespoon per serving)
Prep Time: 15 minutes
Cook Time: 1-2 hours
Total Time: 2-3 hours

Ingredients:

6 large ripe pears (about 3 pounds), peeled, cored, and chopped
1/2 cup apple juice or water
1/2 cup honey or maple syrup (optional, adjust to taste)
1 tablespoon fresh lemon juice
1 vanilla bean, split and seeds scraped (or 1 tablespoon vanilla extract)
1/2 teaspoon ground cinnamon
1/4 teaspoon ground nutmeg
1/4 teaspoon salt

Nutritional Facts (Per Serving):

Calories: 35
Protein: 0g
Carbohydrates: 9g
Dietary Fiber: 1g
Total Sugars: 7g

Preparation

1. Slice the pears into little pieces after peeling and core them. Your pear butter will be sweeter and more delicious the riper the pears are.

2. Prepare the Pears: Put the diced pears, apple juice (or water), and lemon juice in a big saucepan or Dutch oven. Simmer over medium heat for 10 to 15 minutes, or until the pears start to become tender, stirring now and again.

3. Add the spices and sweetener: To the saucepan, add the ground nutmeg, ground cinnamon, ground clover, vanilla bean seeds (or essence), and salt. Mix well to blend.

4. Cook Until It Gets Thick: Turn down the heat to low and simmer the mixture, covered, stirring now and again to avoid sticking. Simmer for one to two hours, or until the stew has thickened enough to spread and the pears are quite tender.

5. Blend until smooth: Take the mixture off of the heat after it has thickened. Puree the mixture with an immersion blender until it's smooth, or move it to a food processor or blender and blend in batches. Leave some pear slices whole if you want your texture chunkier.

6. Modify the consistency and sweetness: Taste the pear butter and add extra honey or maple syrup to suit your taste preference for sweetness. To get the right consistency, thin down any thick parts of the mixture with a little amount of water or apple juice.

7. Hold and Present: Allow the pear butter to reach room temperature. Refrigerate after transferring it to airtight containers or sterilized jars. The pear butter may be canned for extended storage, according to the recommended canning procedures, or kept in the refrigerator for up to two weeks.

8. Serving Ideas: Serve vanilla-pear butter as a topping for porridge or yogurt, or on toast, pancakes, and waffles. It goes well as a stuffing for baked dishes or as an accompaniment to cheese platters.

Warm aromas of vanilla, cinnamon, and nutmeg blend with the sweetness of ripe pears to create a delectably spiced fruit spread known as vanilla-pear butter. It's a wonderful handcrafted present and ideal for a brunch in the autumn or winter.

Recipe 2: Vegan Buffalo Dip

Servings: 8
Prep Time: 10 minutes
Cook Time: 20 minutes

Total Time: 30 minutes

Ingredients:
- 1/2 cups raw cashews, soaked for at least 4 hours or overnight, then drained
- 1/2 cup hot sauce (like Frank's RedHot)
- 1/2 cup unsweetened almond milk or another plant-based milk
- 1/4 cup nutritional yeast
- 1 tablespoon apple cider vinegar
- 1 tablespoon lemon juice
- 1 teaspoon garlic powder
- 1 teaspoon onion powder
- 1/2 teaspoon smoked paprika
- 1/2 teaspoon salt
- 1/2 teaspoon black pepper
- 1 cup canned chickpeas, drained and rinsed, lightly mashed
- 1/2 cup shredded carrots
- 1/2 cup chopped green onions, divided
- 1/4 cup dairy-free shredded cheese (optional)
- 1 tablespoon chopped fresh parsley (optional, for garnish)

Nutritional Facts (Per Serving):
Calories: 190
Protein: 6g
Carbohydrates: 17g
Dietary Fiber: 3g

Total Sugars: 2g
Total Fat: 12g
Saturated Fat: 2g

Preparation

1. Get the cashews ready: To soften the cashews, soak them in water for at least four hours, or overnight. Quick-soak method: Just cover the cashews with boiling water and let them rest for half an hour if you're pressed for time. To use, drain and thoroughly rinse.
2. Mix the Basis: The soaked cashews, spicy sauce, almond milk, nutritional yeast, apple cider vinegar, lemon juice, smoked paprika, garlic powder, onion powder, and salt and black pepper should all be combined in a high-speed blender or food processor. Process the ingredients until it becomes creamy and smooth. One spoonful at a time, add a little more almond milk if it's too thick until you have the right consistency.

Add the veggies and chickpeas and stir.

The blended cashew mixture should be combined with the shredded carrots, half of the chopped green onions, and the gently mashed chickpeas in a mixing dish. Mix everything well by stirring. For added richness, feel free to fold in the shredded dairy-free cheese.

3. Prepare the Dip: Turn the oven on to 375°F, or 190°C. Spoon the mixture into an 8-inch square or comparable ovenproof baking dish. Using a spatula, evenly spread it out. Bake for 20 to 25 minutes, or until the edges of the dip are bubbling hot.

4. Serve and garnish: Take it out of the oven and let it to cool a little. If preferred, garnish with the remaining finely chopped green onions and fresh parsley. Warm up and serve with your favorite dipping foods, such as tortilla chips, carrots, celery sticks, or anything else.

Tips for Storing: For up to five days, leftovers should be kept in the refrigerator in an airtight container. Reheat in the microwave or oven until well heated.

This spicy, creamy, and tasty vegan buffalo dip is great for game days, get-togethers, or as a light snack. This plant-based version is rich in nutrients, dairy-free, and has all the tastes of the traditional dip.

Recipe 3: Chimichurri Sauce

Servings: 8 (2 tablespoons per serving)
Prep Time: 10 minutes
Total Time: 10 minutes

Ingredients:
- 1 cup fresh flat-leaf parsley, finely chopped
- 1/2 cup fresh cilantro, finely chopped (optional)
- 1/4 cup red wine vinegar
- 3-4 garlic cloves, minced
- 1/2 teaspoon crushed red pepper flakes
- 1/2 teaspoon dried oregano
- 1/2 teaspoon salt
- 4 teaspoon black pepper
- 1/2 cup extra-virgin olive oil
- 1 tablespoon fresh lemon juice (optional, for brightness)

Nutritional Facts (Per Serving):
Calories: 120
Protein: 1g
Carbohydrates: 2g
Dietary Fiber: 0.5g
Total Sugars: 0g
Total Fat: 13g
Saturated Fat: 2g

Preparation

1. Cut the Herbs Up: Finely cut the cilantro and fresh parsley, if using. Mince the herbs, but do not purée them. You may use a

food processor, but take care not to grind the ingredients too much—you want a texture that is somewhat grainy.

2.Combine the Base: Chopped parsley, cilantro, minced garlic, dried oregano, crushed red pepper flakes, salt, and black pepper should all be combined in a medium-sized bowl. Mix well by stirring.

3.Include the Liquids: To the herb combination, add the lemon juice (if using) and red wine vinegar. To properly integrate all of the ingredients, slowly pour in the olive oil while swirling constantly. The sauce should be somewhat thick yet properly mixed.

4.Modify the seasoning: After giving the chimichurri a taste, adjust the seasoning by adding additional vinegar, salt, or pepper to your preference. Increase the quantity of crushed red pepper flakes for a hotter variation.

5.Give It a Break: To let the flavors to mingle, let the chimichurri sauce rest at room temperature for at least ten to fifteen minutes. This stage is essential for a taste that is well-rounded.

6. To Serve and Store: Serve the chimichurri sauce as a bread dip or as a garnish for grilled meats and veggies. It's also suitable as a marinade. Any leftovers may be kept in the fridge

for up to a week if they are kept in an airtight container. Before using, give it a good stir.

Chimichurri Sauce is a bright, zesty sauce that enhances any dish with a hint of fresh herbs and goes well with grilled foods. It's easy to prepare, packed with antioxidants and good fats, and a wonderful way to add some color to your meals.

Recipe 4: Creamy Tumeric dressing

Servings: 10 (2 tablespoons per serving)
Prep Time: 10 minutes
Total Time: 10 minutes
Ingredients:
-1/2 cup plain Greek yogurt (or dairy-free yogurt for vegan)
-1/4 cup extra-virgin olive oil
-2 tablespoons apple cider vinegar
-2 tablespoons fresh lemon juice
-1 tablespoon tahini
-2 teaspoons ground turmeric
-1 teaspoon honey or maple syrup (optional, for sweetness)
-1 teaspoon Dijon mustard
-1/2 teaspoon ground cumin
-1/2 teaspoon garlic powder
-1/4 teaspoon salt
-1/4 teaspoon black pepper
-1-2 tablespoons water (optional, to thin if needed)

Nutritional Facts (Per Serving):

Calories: 80

Protein: 1g

Carbohydrates: 2g

Dietary Fiber: 0g

Total Sugars: 1g

Total Fat: 8g

Saturated Fat: 1g

Preparation:

1. Mix the Ingredients Together: Combine the plain Greek yogurt, tahini, apple cider vinegar, extra virgin olive oil, and fresh lemon juice in a medium-sized bowl. Mix until well blended and smooth.

2. Include the Spices: To the bowl, add the powdered turmeric, Dijon mustard, ground cumin, garlic powder, honey (or maple syrup, if using), salt, and black pepper. Repeat whisking until all the ingredients are well combined and the dressing has a smooth, creamy consistency.

3. Modify Coherence: Add 1 to 2 teaspoons of water, one tablespoon at a time, until you have the right consistency if you find that the dressing is too thick. Make sure the water is well mixed in by giving each addition a good whisk.

4.Taste and Modify Seasoning: After tasting the dressing, taste it again and adjust the seasoning by adding additional salt, pepper, or lemon juice to your preferred level.

5.To Serve or Put Away: Serve the creamy turmeric dressing straight away as a dip for fresh vegetables or as a dressing for salads, roasted veggies, and grain bowls. If storing, move the dressing into a sealed jar and keep it in the fridge for a maximum of seven days. The components may separate over time, so thoroughly stir before using each time.

A tasty and nutritious dressing that has anti-inflammatory properties, Creamy Turmeric Dressing gives every meal a blast of flavor and a beautiful golden color. It is very readily veganized and is full of minerals, including the potent antioxidants found in turmeric.

Recipe 5: Strawberry and Chia Seed Jam

Servings: 16 (1 tablespoon per serving)
Prep Time: 10 minutes
Cook Time: 15 minutes
Total Time: 25 minutes

Ingredients:
- 2 cups fresh strawberries, hulled and chopped
- 2 tablespoons maple syrup or honey (optional, adjust to taste)
- 2 tablespoons chia seeds
- 1 tablespoon fresh lemon juice
- 1/2 teaspoon vanilla extract (optional)

Nutritional Facts (Per Serving):
Calories: 15
Protein: 0.5g
Carbohydrates: 3g
Dietary Fiber: 1g
Total Sugars: 1.5g
Total Fat: 0.5g

Preparation

1. Prepare the Strawberries: In a medium saucepan, place the chopped strawberries and heat. Cook, stirring periodically, until the strawberries start to break down and release their juices, approximately 5 to 7 minutes. The back of a spoon or a potato masher may be used to assist mash the strawberries to the proper consistency.

2. Enhance the Jam's Taste: Pour in the honey or maple syrup (if using) into the pot. Mix well to blend. Based on your own

preference and the strawberries' inherent sweetness, adjust the sweetness.

3. Thicken with Chia Seeds Added: Add the lemon juice and chia seeds and stir. Stirring constantly, continue heating the mixture for an additional five to seven minutes, or until the jam starts to thicken. The chia seeds will naturally thicken the jam by absorbing the liquid and forming a gel-like structure.

4. Complete the Jam: After taking the pot off of the burner, mix in the vanilla essence, if using. Give the jam ten minutes or so to cool. It will continue to thicken as it cools.

5. Hold and Present: Spoon the jam into an airtight jar or clean glass jar. Allow it to cool fully before capping the container. The jam may be kept in the fridge for one to two weeks. Although the jam may be used right away, it tastes best when served after chilling for a few hours to let the flavors combine.

6. Serving Ideas: Savor this delightful and nutritious Strawberry and Chia Seed Jam as a topping for sweets or as an addition to toast, porridge, yogurt, and pancakes. It works well as a filling for baked products and as an addition to smoothies.

A simple, nutrient-dense, refined sugar-free substitute for typical jams is strawberry and chia seed jam. Because chia seeds are high in fiber, antioxidants, and omega-3 fatty acids, this jam is not only delicious but healthy as well.

Recipe 6: Caramelized onions

Servings: 8 (1/4 cup per serving)
Prep Time: 10 minutes
Cook Time: 45 minutes
Total Time: 55 minutes

Ingredients:
- 4 large yellow onions, thinly sliced (about 6 cups)
- 2 tablespoons extra-virgin olive oil
- 1 tablespoon unsalted butter (optional, for richer flavor
- 1/2 teaspoon salt
- 1/2 teaspoon sugar (optional, to aid in caramelization)
- 1/4 cup water or vegetable broth (if needed)

Nutritional Facts (Per Serving):
Calories: 70
Protein: 1g
Carbohydrates: 9g
Dietary Fiber: 1.5g
Total Sugars: 4g
Total Fat: 4g
Saturated Fat: 1g

Preparation

1.Get the onions ready: After peeling, split the onions in half. Cut each half into half-moons with a thin slice. The slices will caramelize more quickly if they are thinner.

2.Warm up the pan: Melt and shimmer the butter, if using, and olive oil in a large skillet or heavy-based pan over medium heat. Use simply olive oil for a vegan version if you'd choose.

3.Include the onions: Spread out the onions after adding them to the pan in slices. For more moisture wicking and caramelization, lightly dust with sugar and salt, if using. Coat the onions well with the oil and butter mixture by stirring.

4.Make the Onions Caramel: Cook the onions steadily over medium-low heat, stirring them every few minutes. The onions will release their natural sugars and begin to take on a golden brown color as they cook. Approximately 30 to 45 minutes are needed for this procedure, depending on the desired amount of caramelization. Reduce the heat quickly to prevent burning instead of caramelizing; alternatively, take your time.

5. Clear the Pan: Deglaze the pan by adding a little amount of water or vegetable broth, one to two teaspoons at a time, if the onions begin to cling to the bottom. This will add depth of flavor

by loosening any browned pieces that have adhered to the bottom. Stirring constantly, cook until the liquid is gone.

6. Verify whether it's done: When the onions are tender, their color deep golden brown, and their taste rich and sweet, they are done. If necessary, add extra salt to the seasoning after tasting it.

Hold and Present: After taking the caramelized onions off of the stove, let them to cool somewhat. Add them right away to soups, stews, or dips, or use them as a topping for sandwiches, burgers, and steaks. Remaining food may be refrigerated for up to five days in an airtight container or frozen for up to three months.

Rich, salty, and sweet flavors are added to many meals with great success when onions are caramelized. Using a few basic ingredients and perseverance, you can turn regular onions into a tasty and versatile ingredient.

Recipe 7: Tangy Barbecue sauce with Apple Cider vinegar

Servings: 16 (2 tablespoons per serving)
Prep Time: 5 minutes
Cook Time: 20 minutes
Total Time: 25 minutes

Ingredients:
- 1 cup tomato sauce (or ketchup for a sweeter base)
- 1/2 cup apple cider vinegar
- 1/4 cup molasses
- 1/4 cup maple syrup or honey
- 2 tablespoons Worcestershire sauce (use vegan **Worcestershire sauce for a vegan version**)
- 1 tablespoon Dijon mustard
- 1 tablespoon smoked paprika
- 1 teaspoon garlic powder
- 1 teaspoon onion powder
- 1/2 teaspoon cayenne pepper (optional, for heat)
- 1/2 teaspoon salt
- 1/4 teaspoon black pepper
- 1 tablespoon liquid smoke (optional, for smokiness)

Nutritional Facts (Per Serving):
Calories: 40
Protein: 0.5g
Carbohydrates: 10g
Dietary Fiber: 0.5g
Total Sugars: 8g

Preparation

1. Mix the Basic Ingredients together: The apple cider vinegar, molasses, tomato sauce (or ketchup), and maple syrup (or honey) should all be combined in a medium pot. Mix until well blended and smooth.

2. Include the seasonings: To the pot, add the Worcestershire sauce, Dijon mustard, smoked paprika, onion and garlic powders, cayenne (if using), salt, and black pepper. To mix in all the ingredients, whisk the sauce one more.

3. Reduce the Heat in the Sauce: After setting the pot on medium heat, carefully simmer the mixture. Turn down the heat to low and simmer, stirring now and again, for around 15 to 20 minutes. This allows the sauce to gradually thicken and the flavors to mingle. Add liquid smoke during the final five minutes of cooking if using.

4. Modify Coherence: Simmer the sauce until it reaches the consistency you wish, if you like it thicker. Add a little bit of water, one tablespoon at a time, to the sauce if it becomes too thick, and whisk until the right consistency is achieved.

5. Taste and Modify Seasoning: After tasting the sauce, taste again and adjust the seasoning by adding additional sugar, salt, or pepper to your taste. Increase the apple cider vinegar a little bit for a tangier sauce.

6. Chill and Store: After taking the sauce off the stove, let it to reach room temperature. Move it into an airtight jar or clean glass jar. The sauce may be kept for up to two weeks in the refrigerator. Before using, give it a good shake or mix, since separation might happen.

7. Serving Ideas: This zesty barbecue sauce may be used as a basting sauce for chicken, tofu, or grilled veggies as well as a marinade for meats. It's also delicious on sandwiches and as a burger topper.

For those who want a little tang in their BBQ, our Tangy BBQ Sauce with Apple Cider Vinegar is ideal. A well-balanced and savory sauce is produced by the combination of the sour taste of apple cider vinegar with the depth and sweetness of molasses and maple syrup.

Recipe 8: Old-fashioned Applesauce

Servings: 8 (1/2 cup per serving)
Prep Time: 10 minutes
Cook Time: 25 minutes
Total Time: 35 minutes

Ingredients:

- 6 medium apples (about 2 pounds), peeled, cored, and chopped (preferably a mix of sweet and tart apples, like Granny Smith, Honeycrisp, or Fuji)
- 1/2 cup water
- 1-2 tablespoons lemon juice
- 2 tablespoons maple syrup or honey (optional, adjust to taste)
- 1 teaspoon ground cinnamon (optional)
- 1/4 teaspoon ground nutmeg (optional)
- 1/4 teaspoon salt

Nutritional Facts (Per Serving):

Calories: 70
Protein: 0.3g
Carbohydrates: 18g
Dietary Fiber: 3g
Total Sugars: 14g
Total Fat: 0g

Preparation:

1. Get the apples ready: Apples should be peeled, cored, and chopped into tiny pieces. The final applesauce's texture will depend on the size of the pieces; chop bigger pieces for a chunkier sauce.

2.Prepare the Apples: Put the chopped apples, water, and lemon juice in a big pot or saucepan. Lemon juice gives the apples a little brightness in taste and keeps them from browning.

3.Add the spices and sweetener: To the saucepan, add the ground nutmeg, ground cinnamon, and ground maple syrup (or honey, if using). Mix all the ingredients well by stirring.

4.Simmer to Make Soft: Heat the mixture on medium-high and bring it to a boil. After it boils, lower the heat to a simmer, cover, and let it cook for 20 to 25 minutes while stirring from time to time. Cook the apples until they are very tender and easily mashed with a fork or spoon.

5.Blend or mash the apple sauce: Use a potato masher to mash the softened apples to the appropriate consistency if you want a chunky applesauce. Use an immersion blender or transfer to a blender and purée until smooth for a smoother sauce. When combining hot liquids, use caution.

6.Chill and Store: To bring the applesauce to room temperature, let it cool. Pour it into sealed jars or clean glass jars. You may freeze it for up to three months or keep it in the fridge for up to one week.

7.Serving Ideas: Savor this classic applesauce as a snack on its own or as an accompaniment to roasted meats, pork chops, pancakes, or yogurt. It works well as a basis for baking and in certain recipes as an alternative to sugar or fat.

A traditional dish that is easy to make, naturally sweet, and soothing is Old-Fashioned Applesauce. This is a delicious and adaptable condiment that combines tart and sweet apples with a touch of nutmeg and cinnamon.

Recipe 9: Avocado -Dill Sauce

Servings: 8 (2 tablespoons per serving)
Prep Time: 10 minutes
Total Time: 10 minutes

Ingredients:
-1 large ripe avocado, peeled, pitted, and chopped
-1/2 cup plain Greek yogurt (or dairy-free yogurt for a vegan option)
-2 tablespoons fresh lemon juice
-2 tablespoons fresh dill, chopped
-1 clove garlic, minced
-1 tablespoon extra-virgin olive oil
-1/4 teaspoon salt
-1/4 teaspoon black pepper
-2-3 tablespoons water (to thin, as needed)

Nutritional Facts (Per Serving):
Calories: 60
Protein: 1g
Carbohydrates: 3g
Dietary Fiber: 1g
Total Sugars: 0.5g
Total Fat: 5g
Saturated Fat: 1g

Preparation

1. Get the ingredients ready: Cut the avocado into pieces after peeling and pitting it. Chop the fresh dill and mince the garlic. Put aside.

2. In a blender, combine the ingredients: Add the chopped avocado, plain Greek yogurt, extra-virgin olive oil, minced garlic, fresh lemon juice, fresh dill, salt, and black pepper to a blender or food processor.

3. Blend until smooth: Process the sauce on high until it becomes creamy and smooth. Add water one tablespoon at a time to the mixture if it's too thick until you have the right consistency. Not too runny, but just smooth enough to use.

4.Taste and Modify Seasoning: After tasting the sauce, taste it again and adjust the seasoning by adding additional salt, pepper, or lemon juice to your preference.

5.To Serve or Put Away: Serve the Avocado-Dill Sauce right away as a dressing, dip, or sauce after transferring it to a bowl. If keeping, keep it in the refrigerator for up to three days in an airtight container. Press a piece of plastic wrap directly across the sauce's surface before closing it to stop it from browning.

6.Serving Ideas: This sauce is delicious on salads, grain bowls, grilled chicken, seafood, and as a spread on wraps and sandwiches.

A creamy, savory, and refreshing complement to many foods is avocado-dill sauce. Richness and tanginess are well balanced by the addition of fresh dill, avocado, garlic, and lemon. Ideal for a flexible and healthful sauce!

Recipe 10: Garden Marinara sauce

Servings: 8 (1/2 cup per serving)
Prep Time: 15 minutes
Cook Time: 30 minutes
Total Time: 45 minutes

Ingredients:
- 2 tablespoons extra-virgin olive oil
- 1 large onion, finely chopped
- 4 cloves garlic, minced
- 2 medium carrots, finely chopped
- 2 stalks celery, finely chopped
- 1 large red bell pepper, finely chopped
- 1 medium zucchini, finely chopped
- 1 (28-ounce) can crushed tomatoes
- 1 (15-ounce) can diced tomatoes
- 1/4 cup tomato paste
- 1/2 cup fresh basil leaves, chopped (or 1 tablespoon dried basil)
- 1 tablespoon dried oregano
- 1/2 teaspoon red pepper flakes (optional, for heat)
- 1 teaspoon salt
- 1/2 teaspoon black pepper
- 1 teaspoon sugar (optional, to balance acidity)
- 1/4 cup fresh parsley, chopped

Nutritional Facts (Per Serving):
Calories: 90
Protein: 2g
Carbohydrates: 12g
Dietary Fiber: 3g
Total Sugars: 6g
Total Fat: 4g
Saturated Fat: 0.5g

Preparation:

1. Get the veggies ready: Chop the zucchini, red bell pepper, carrots, celery, and onion finely. Dice the garlic. Put aside.

2. Cook the Veggies: In a big saucepan or Dutch oven, warm the olive oil over medium heat. When the onion is tender and transparent, add it and sauté it for three to four minutes. Add the red bell pepper, zucchini, carrots, celery, and garlic. Simmer the veggies for a further five to seven minutes, stirring now and again, until they are tender.

3. Include the Herbs and Tomatoes: To the saucepan, add the tomato paste, diced tomatoes, and crushed tomatoes. Mix well to blend. Add the sugar (if used), salt, black pepper, dried oregano, red pepper flakes (if using), and chopped basil. Stir one more to fully combine all the ingredients.

4. Reduce the Heat in the Sauce: Over medium-high heat, bring the mixture to a boil and then turn down the heat. Allow the sauce to simmer, covered, for twenty to twenty-five minutes, stirring now and again to help the flavors combine and avoid sticking.

5. Modify the Seasoning: After tasting the sauce, taste again and adjust the seasoning by adding additional salt, pepper, or herbs to suit your taste.

6. Lastly, add some fresh herbs: During the last five minutes of cooking, stir in the chopped fresh parsley to add fresh herbs and improve the taste.

7. To Serve or Put Away: After taking the sauce off the stove, let it to cool somewhat. Serve right away with your favorite Italian foods, spaghetti, or as a pizza sauce. Alternatively, allow it to cool fully before transferring it to sealed jars. You may freeze it for up to three months or keep it in the fridge for up to five days.

8. Serving Ideas: Use this Garden Marinara Sauce as the foundation for lasagna, as a dip for breadsticks, as a grilled chicken or eggplant topping, or combined with other ingredients to make a grain or vegetable bowl.

Packed with fresh vegetables and herbs, Garden Marinara Sauce adds flavor and nutrition to every dish. It's a wonderful way to savor a thick, flavorful sauce that has plenty of natural sweetness and little added sugar.

Chapter 4: Plant-Based Mains

Mains Based on Plants: Eating more plant-based foods may have significant anti-inflammatory effects on your body. Whole, plant-based diets are high in fiber, healthy fats, and antioxidants that help reduce inflammation in the body. This area offers a selection of tasty, high-nutrient plant-based main courses that are ideal for anybody trying to enhance their general health, decrease inflammation, and increase energy.

Fresh veggies, legumes, whole grains, nuts, seeds, and healthy oils are the main ingredients in these recipes, which combine to provide tasty, filling meals that will keep you feeling full and energetic all day. These recipes are meant to be tasty and easy to make, regardless of whether you are a dedicated plant-based eater or just want to include more plant-based meals in your diet.

The following are some of the main anti-inflammatory ingredients found in plant-based meals: - Leafy Greens (Kale, Spinach, Swiss Chard):Rich in antioxidants, fiber, and vitamins A, C, and K, these foods also assist to decrease inflammation. Brussels sprouts, cauliflower, and broccoli are examples of cruciferous vegetables that have sulforaphane, a substance that may help lessen inflammation.

Whole Grains (Brown Rice, Quinoa, and Farro): Packed with fiber, vitamins, and minerals, these grains help to lower inflammation and promote intestinal health.
- Legumes (Black beans, chickpeas, and lentils):High in fiber, protein, and phytochemicals that reduce inflammation.

-Nuts and seeds (flaxseeds, chia seeds, and walnuts): Rich in omega-3 fatty acids, which have anti-inflammatory qualities.

- Herbs and Spices (Garlic, Ginger, Turmeric, and Basil): These ingredients have strong anti-inflammatory properties and flavor food without adding too much sugar or salt.
- Healthy Fats (extra-virgin olive oil, avocado): Offer monounsaturated fats that lower inflammation and promote heart health.

Recommended Recipes:

1. Vegetable Stir-Fry with Ginger-Turmeric Sauce for Chickpeas
- A vibrant, nutrient-dense stir-fry with snap peas, bell peppers, zucchini, and chickpeas combined with a ginger-turmeric sauce that enhances its anti-inflammatory properties. For a full dinner, serve over quinoa or brown rice.

2. Bento Bowl with Quinoa and Sweet Potato, Roasted sweet potatoes, steaming kale, chickpeas, and protein-rich quinoa are all combined in this filling dish and dressed with a creamy tahini sauce. It has a ton of fiber, antioxidants, and good fats to promote general health and lower inflammation.

3. Spunky and Lentil Filled Bell Peppers

 - Baked till soft, bell peppers are packed with a flavorful blend of green lentils, spinach, tomatoes, garlic, and herbs. This meal is high in fiber, protein, and anti-inflammatory vitamins A and C.

4. Curried Chickpeas with Cauliflower: Curry prepared with cauliflower, chickpeas, tomatoes, and spinach that is served warm and is flavored with turmeric, cumin, coriander, and ginger in a fragrant coconut milk sauce. Serve with whole-grain naan or brown rice for a warming, anti-inflammatory supper.

5. Tomato and Herb Stuffed Eggplant with Mediterranean Flavor: After roasting, eggplants are filled with a tasty mixture of chickpeas, tomatoes, parsley, and pine nuts that has been seasoned with extra virgin olive oil, garlic, and lemon. A full yet light supper option, this meal is delicious.

6. Mushroom and Lentil Shepherd's Pie: An alternative comfort food made with plants. A low-carb, anti-inflammatory substitute

for conventional potatoes, this shepherd's pie has a delicious foundation of mushrooms, lentils, carrots, and peas, topped with creamy mashed cauliflower.

7. Zucchini Noodles with Cherry Tomatoes and Avocado Pesto: A light and refreshing meal with spiralized zucchini noodles combined with pine nuts, juicy cherry tomatoes, and a creamy avocado pesto sauce. This recipe is a great source of antioxidants, fiber, and healthy fats.

8. Spicy Enchiladas with Sweet Potato and Black Beans: A homemade tomato-based enchilada sauce is served on top of these enchiladas, which are packed with a flavorful mixture of sweet potatoes, onions, black beans, and spices. Perfectly baked, they come with a side of avocado and lime.

9. Quinoa Stuffed Acorn Squash with Roasted Veggies: After roasting until soft, quinoa, roasted veggies, cranberries, and walnuts are filled into acorn squash. This recipe is ideal for an anti-inflammatory, warming, and nutrient-dense supper.

10. Veggie and Chickpea Stew with Golden Flavor: A filling and dense stew with coconut milk, kale, carrots, potatoes, and chickpeas that is flavored with ginger, cumin, and turmeric, which have anti-inflammatory properties. Serve this dish with some crusty whole-grain bread for a hearty and filling dinner.

These colorful, tasty, and bursting with anti-inflammatory components plant-based main meals are meant to be enjoyed by everybody. With so many alternatives for every occasion and dietary requirement, these dishes are perfect for a simple weekday supper or a more extravagant feast to wow visitors. Savor the advantages of a plant-based diet and discover the deliciousness of anti-inflammatory food!

To help readers prepare tasty, healthful meals, this section offers a wide range of plant-based main dishes, each highlighting anti-inflammatory elements.

Recipe1 : White Beans and French Onions Soup

Servings: 6

Prep Time: 15 minutes
Cook Time: 45 minutes
Total Time: 1 hour

Ingredients:
-3 tablespoons extra-virgin olive oil
-4 large yellow onions, thinly sliced
-4 cloves garlic, minced
-1 tablespoon fresh thyme leaves (or 1 teaspoon dried thyme)
-1 tablespoon balsamic vinegar
-1/2 cup dry white wine (optional)
-4 cups low-sodium vegetable broth
-2 cups water
-2 (15-ounce) cans white beans (cannellini or Great Northern beans), drained and rinsed
-1 bay leaf
-1 teaspoon salt
-1/2 teaspoon black pepper
-1/4 teaspoon red pepper flakes (optional)
-1/2 cup fresh parsley, chopped (for garnish)
-Whole-grain or gluten-free baguette slices, toasted (optional)

Nutritional Facts (Per Serving):

Calories: 180

Protein: 5g

Carbohydrates: 25g

Dietary Fiber: 5g

Total Sugars: 6g

Total Fat: 7g

Saturated Fat: 1g

Preparation

1. Make the Onions Caramel: In a big saucepan or Dutch oven, warm the olive oil over medium heat. After adding the onions, slice them and simmer for 20 to 25 minutes, stirring now and again, until they are fully caramelized and golden brown. To deglaze and keep the onions from burning, add a dash of water if they begin to cling to the bottom of the saucepan.

2. Add the thyme and garlic: Add the chopped garlic and thyme leaves and stir. Cook the garlic for one to two minutes, or until fragrant.

3. Use wine and balsamic vinegar to deglaze: After scraping away any browned parts from the bottom of the saucepan, add the balsamic vinegar to the pot. If using white wine, add it now and

boil for two to three minutes to reduce the alcohol and improve the taste.

4. Add the beans, water, and broth: Add the white beans and bay leaf after adding the water and vegetable broth. Mix well to blend.

5. Reduce the Soup's Heat: Over medium-high heat, bring the soup to a boil and then turn down the heat. To let the flavors to merge together, cover and simmer for 20 to 25 minutes.

6. Add flavor to the soup: After removing the bay leaf, add salt, black pepper, and (if preferred) red pepper flakes to the soup. Adjust the seasoning according to your taste.

7. Present the Soup: Spoon the heated soup into individual bowls and top with freshly chopped parsley. If preferred, provide with slices of gluten-free or whole-grain bread on the side.

8. Decorative Accents Not Required: Add a piece of bread to the top of each dish and some vegan or dairy-free cheese for an added touch. For a really warming ending, broil the cheese until it is melted and bubbling.

A filling and cozy food that provides a healthy balance of fiber, protein, and taste is white beans and french onion soup. It's ideal for a comforting dinner that promotes a diet low in inflammation.

Recipe 2: Masala Lentil

Servings: 4
Prep Time: 10 minutes
Cook Time: 30 minutes
Total Time: 40 minutes

Ingredients:
-1 cup dried red lentils, rinsed
-2 tablespoons extra-virgin olive oil or coconut oil
-1 large onion, finely chopped
-3 cloves garlic, minced
-1 tablespoon fresh ginger, minced
-2 teaspoons ground cumin
-1 teaspoon ground coriander
-1 teaspoon ground turmeric
-1/2 teaspoon ground cinnamon
-1/4 teaspoon cayenne pepper (optional)
-1 (14-ounce) can diced tomatoes
-1 (14-ounce) can coconut milk (full fat or light)
-2 cups low-sodium vegetable broth
-1 teaspoon salt
-1/2 teaspoon black pepper
-1/4 cup fresh cilantro, chopped (for garnish)
-Juice of 1/2 lemon
-Cooked brown rice or quinoa (for serving, optional)

Nutritional Facts (Per Serving):
Calories: 320
Protein: 13g
Carbohydrates: 40g
Dietary Fiber: 13g
Total Sugars: 5g
Total Fat: 13g
Saturated Fat: 7g

Preparation

1. Aromatics in sauté: In a large saucepan set over medium heat, warm the coconut oil or olive oil. When the onion is tender and transparent, add it and sauté it for five to six minutes. When aromatic, add the minced garlic and ginger and simmer for an additional one to two minutes.

2. Include Spices: Toss in the turmeric, ground cumin, coriander, cinnamon, and cayenne (if using). After thoroughly stirring to coat the onions, heat for one to two minutes to toast the spices and release their scent.

3. Add the broth, tomatoes, and lentils: To the saucepan, add the chopped tomatoes, vegetable broth, and rinsed lentils. Toss to thoroughly mix in all the ingredients. Heat the mixture on medium-high and bring it to a boil.

4. Reduce the heat of the lentils: After lowering the heat to low and covering the pot, simmer the lentils for around 20 minutes, stirring from time to time, or until they become soft and the flavors combine. As necessary, add a bit more vegetable broth or water if the mixture becomes too thick.

5. Season and add the coconut milk: To make the soup creamy and to enable the flavors to mingle, stir in the coconut milk and simmer for an additional five minutes. To taste, add a squeeze of lemon juice, salt, and black pepper.

6. Serve: Spoon the Masala Lentil mixture into individual bowls and sprinkle with finely chopped cilantro. Serve hot for a filling and full dinner over cooked quinoa or brown rice.

7. Decorative Accents Not Required: For extra texture and taste, top with a dollop of dairy-free yogurt or a scattering of toasted nuts or seeds.

An anti-inflammatory diet would benefit greatly from the tasty and nutrient-dense meal called masala lentil. Spices, lentils, and coconut milk come together to create a filling, cozy, and robust dish that is high in fiber and plant-based protein. Savor this recipe as a side dish to go with other foods or as a main course with rice.

Recipe 3: Minestrone Soup

Servings: 6
Prep Time: 15 minutes
Cook Time: 30 minutes
Total Time: 45 minutes

Ingredients:
- 2 tablespoons extra-virgin olive oil
- 1 large onion, diced
- 3 cloves garlic, minced
- 2 medium carrots, diced
- 2 celery stalks, diced
- 1 red bell pepper, diced
- 1 zucchini, diced
- 1 cup green beans, chopped
- 1 (14-ounce) can diced tomatoes
- 1 (15-ounce) can kidney beans, drained and rinsed
- 1 cup frozen peas
- 4 cups low-sodium vegetable broth
- 2 cups water
- 1 teaspoon dried basil
- 1 teaspoon dried oregano
- 1/2 teaspoon dried thyme
- 1 bay leaf
- 1 teaspoon salt

- 1/2 teaspoon black pepper
- 1 cup whole-grain pasta or gluten-free pasta (optional)
- 1/4 cup fresh parsley, chopped (for garnish)
- Juice of 1/2 lemon (optional)

Nutritional Facts (Per Serving):
Calories: 220
Protein: 9g
Carbohydrates: 36g
Dietary Fiber: 8g
Total Sugars: 8g
Total Fat: 7g
Saturated Fat: 1g

Preparation

1. Cook the Veggies: In a big saucepan or Dutch oven, warm the olive oil over medium heat. Add the celery, carrots, and chopped onion. After the veggies are softened, sauté them for five to seven minutes. Cook for a further one to two minutes after adding the minced garlic.

2. Add the green beans, zucchini, and bell pepper: Add the chopped green beans, chopped zucchini, and diced red bell pepper. Cook until the veggies are slightly soft, about 5 more minutes.

3. Add the beans and tomatoes: Stir in the kidney beans, frozen peas, and chopped tomatoes. Mix well to blend.

4. Add the herbs, water, and broth: Add the water and veggie broth. Add the black pepper, salt, bay leaf, oregano, thyme, and dried basil. Mix everything well with a stir.

5. Reduce the Soup's Heat: After bringing the soup to a boil, turn down the heat. Once the flavors have combined and the veggies are soft, cover and simmer for 15 to 20 minutes.

6. Pasta Cooking (Optional): If using pasta, toss it into the soup and cook it for the amount of time specified on the box, generally 8 to 10 minutes, or until it's al dente.

7. Complete and Present: From the soup, remove the bay leaf. If necessary, adjust the seasoning by adding more salt and pepper. Just before serving, stir in the fresh parsley and squeeze of lemon juice (if using).

8. Serve: Spoon heated minestrone soup into individual dishes. Savor it on its own or as a whole meal with a side of whole-grain bread.

A filling, nutrient-dense food ideal for an anti-inflammatory diet is minestrone soup. Tightly packed with an assortment of veggies, beans, and herbs, it provides a hearty, high-fiber, and vitamin-rich meal with a rich taste profile.

Recipe 4: Jam-packed Pepper

Servings: 4
Prep Time: 15 minutes
Cook Time: 35 minutes
Total Time: 50 minutes

Ingredients:
-4 large bell peppers (red, yellow, or green)
-1 tablespoon extra-virgin olive oil
-1 medium onion, diced
-2 cloves garlic, minced
-1 cup cooked quinoa or brown
-1 (15-ounce) can black beans, drained and rinsed
-1 cup corn kernels (fresh, frozen, or canned)
-1 medium tomato, diced
-1/2 cup diced zucchini
-1/2 cup shredded carrots
-1/2 cup low-sodium vegetable broth
-1 teaspoon ground cumin
-1 teaspoon smoked paprika
-1/2 teaspoon chili powder
-1/2 teaspoon salt

-1/4 teaspoon black pepper
-1/2 cup shredded dairy-free cheese (optional)
-1/4 cup fresh cilantro, chopped (for garnish)
-1 tablespoon lime juice (optional)

Nutritional Facts (Per Serving):
Calories: 250
Protein: 8g
Carbohydrates: 45g
Dietary Fiber: 11g
Total Sugars: 6g
Total Fat: 5g
Saturated Fat: 1g

Preparation

1. Turn the oven on to 375°F (190°C) and prepare the peppers. Remove the seeds and membranes from the bell peppers by slicing off the tops. Put the peppers away.

2. Sauté Vegetables: Place a large skillet over medium heat with the olive oil. Add the diced onion and cook, stirring, until it becomes soft, about 5 minutes. When the garlic is fragrant, add the minced garlic and cook for an extra minute.

3. Put the remaining veggies and spices in the skillet: Add the black beans, corn, shredded carrots, diced tomato, and zucchini. Toss to mix thoroughly. Incorporate the cooked brown rice or

quinoa, smoked paprika, chili powder, ground cumin, black pepper, and salt. Cook, stirring occasionally, until the mixture is thoroughly heated and well combined, 5 to 7 minutes.

4. Fill the Peppers to the Brim: Tightly pack and fill each bell pepper with the quinoa and vegetable mixture, using a spoon. Arrange the filled peppers, standing straight, in a baking dish. Top each pepper with shredded dairy-free cheese if you'd like.

5. Bake the Peppers: Bake the baking dish in the preheated oven for twenty-five minutes, covered with aluminum foil. After ten more minutes, or until the peppers are soft and the tops are beginning to brown, remove the foil and continue baking.

6. Garnish and Serve: Take the stuffed peppers out of the oven and let them a few minutes to cool before serving. If preferred, garnish with freshly chopped cilantro and a squeeze of lime juice. Warm servings are recommended.

A meal that is bright, nutrient-dense, and full, Jam-Packed Pepper is an excellent choice for a diet that is designed to reduce inflammation. A nutritious mix of fiber, protein, and important nutrients may be obtained by consuming a variety of whole grains, beans, and fresh vegetables. It is a recipe that may be modified to suit the kind of components that are readily accessible or to suit the preferences of the individual.

Recipe 5: Wild rice Soup with Mushrooms

Servings: 6
Prep Time: 15 minutes
Cook Time: 45 minutes
Total Time: 1 hour

Ingredients:
-1 cup wild rice, rinsed
-2 tablespoons extra-virgin olive oil
-1 large onion, diced
-3 cloves garlic, minced
-2 medium carrots, diced
celery stalks, diced
-12 ounces mushrooms (such as cremini, button, or shiitake), sliced
-1 teaspoon dried thyme
-1 teaspoon dried rosemary
-1/2 teaspoon dried sage
-1/4 teaspoon crushed red pepper flakes (optional)
-4 cups low-sodium vegetable broth
-2 cups water
-1 (14-ounce) can full-fat coconut
-2 tablespoons cornstarch or arrowroot powder (optional, for thickening)
-1 teaspoon salt
-1/2 teaspoon black pepper
-2 tablespoons fresh parsley, chopped (for garnish)

-Juice of 1/2 lemon (optional, for added brightness)

Nutritional Facts (Per Serving):
Calories: 250
Protein: 5g
Carbohydrates: 31g
Dietary Fiber: 4g
Total Sugars: 4g
Total Fat: 13g

Preparation

1. Prepare the Wild Rice: Three cups of water and the washed wild rice should be combined in a medium pot. Heat to a boil on a medium-high heat setting. Once the rice is soft and has absorbed the majority of the water, reduce the heat to low, cover, and simmer for 40 to 45 minutes. After the rice has cooked, drain any extra water and put it aside.

2. Quickly sauté the veggies: In a big saucepan or Dutch oven set over medium heat, warm the olive oil while the rice is cooking. Add the chopped onion, carrots, and celery. To soften the veggies, sauté them for about 5 to 6 minutes. Sauté the minced garlic for one further minute, or until it begins to release its aroma.

3. Get the Mushrooms Cooked: Add the sliced mushrooms to the saucepan and simmer for 5-7 minutes until they are browned and have shed their liquid. Stir periodically to avoid sticking.

4. Add Herbs and Broth: Stir in the dried thyme, rosemary, sage, and crushed red pepper flakes (if using). Cook for 1 minute to unleash their flavors. Pour in the veggie broth and 2 cups of water. Bring the soup to a boil, then decrease the heat to low and let it simmer for 10 minutes.

5. Add Coconut Milk and Thicken (if desired): Stir in the full-fat coconut milk and continue to cook for another 5 minutes. If you like a thicker soup, combine 2 teaspoons of cornstarch or arrowroot powder with 2 tablespoons of water to produce a slurry, then add it to the pot. Cook for a further 2-3 minutes, stirring regularly until the soup thickens.

6. Incorporate the cooked wild rice: Add the black pepper, salt, and cooked wild rice and stir. To let the flavors mingle, boil the soup for a further five minutes.

7. Complete and Present: Take the soup off the stove and, to enliven the tastes, toss in some fresh parsley and, if desired, a squeeze of lemon juice. If necessary, taste and add additional salt or pepper to the seasoning.

8.Serve: Serve the heated Wild Rice Soup with Mushrooms warm by ladling it into bowls. It tastes great served with a crisp green salad or with some crusty whole-grain bread.

An anti-inflammatory diet would benefit greatly from this creamy, satisfying, and filling meal of wild rice soup with mushrooms. A filling dish full of fiber, vitamins, and minerals is created when wild rice, mushrooms, and fragrant herbs are combined.

Recipe 6: Balsamic Beet

Servings: 4
Prep Time: 10 minutes
Cook Time: 45 minutes
Total Time: 55 minutes

Ingredients:
-4 medium beets, scrubbed and trimmed
-2 tablespoons extra-virgin olive oil
-2 tablespoons balsamic vinegar
-1 tablespoon honey ormaple syrup
-1 teaspoon Dijon mustard
-1/2 teaspoon salt
-1/4 teaspoon black pepper
-1 tablespoon fresh parsley, chopped (for garnish)
-1 tablespoon crumbled goat cheese or vegan cheese (optional)

Nutritional Facts (Per Serving):
Calories: 120
Protein: 2g
Carbohydrates: 16g
Dietary Fiber: 4g
Total Sugars: 12g
Total Fat: 6g
Saturated Fat: 1g

Preparation

1. Roast and prepare the beetsSet oven temperature to 400°F, or 200°C. Place the individual beets on a baking sheet, each wrapped in aluminum foil. When a fork pierces the beets, they are done. Roast in the preheated oven for 40 to 45 minutes. The size of the beets will determine how long they need to cook.

2. For the Balsamic Glaze, prepare: Make the balsamic glaze while the beets roast. Mix the olive oil, balsamic vinegar, honey (or maple syrup), Dijon mustard, salt, and black pepper in a small bowl until well blended. Put aside.

3. Slice and peel the beets: After the beets are done, take them out of the oven and let them to cool down for a little while until they become manageable. Strip the beets' skins using a paper towel. As an alternative, you may use a tiny paring knife to take

off the skin. Cut the beets into rounds or wedges that are 1/4 inch thick.

4.Assemble the Beets: The sliced beets should be put in a serving dish. After making the balsamic glaze, drizzle it over the beets and toss them slightly to ensure that the dressing coats them evenly.

5.Serve and garnish: For extra taste and texture, garnish with finely chopped parsley and crumbled goat cheese or vegan cheese, if using. Serve as a light salad or as a side dish, heated or room temperature.

A tasty and nutrient-dense side dish that is ideal for an anti-inflammatory diet is balsamic beets. The tart balsamic glaze brings out the natural sweetness of the roasted beets, making this a tasty and nutritious side dish for any occasion. In addition to being high in fiber, vitamins, and minerals, this meal is a wonderful way to savor the earthy beet tastes.

Recipe 7:Indian -Spice Cauliflower

Servings: 4
Prep Time: 10 minutes
Cook Time: 25 minutes
Total Time: 35 minutes

Ingredients:
- 1 large head of cauliflower, cut into florets
- 2 tablespoons extra-virgin olive oil
- 1 teaspoon ground turmeric
- 1 teaspoon ground cumin
- 1 teaspoon ground coriander
- 1/2 teaspoon ground paprika
- 1/2 teaspoon garam masala
- 1/4 teaspoon ground cayenne pepper (optional, for heat)
- 1/2 teaspoon salt
- 1/4 teaspoon black pepper
- 1 tablespoon lemon juice
- 2 tablespoons fresh cilantro, chopped (for garnish)
- 1 tablespoon sesame seeds (optional, for garnish)

Nutritional Facts (Per Serving):
Calories: 110
Protein: 3g
Carbohydrates: 10g
Dietary Fiber: 4g
Total Sugars: 3g
Total Fat: 7g
Saturated Fat: 1g

Preparation

1. Warm up the oven: Set the oven temperature to 425°F (220°C). A large baking sheet may be gently oiled with olive oil or lined with parchment paper.

Get the spice mixture ready. Combine the turmeric, cumin, coriander, paprika, garam masala, salt, black pepper, and cayenne (if using) in a small bowl.

2. How to season cauliflower: Place the cauliflower florets in a large mixing basin. Pour in a little olive oil and stir to ensure uniform coating. To make sure every floret of cauliflower is well covered in the spices, sprinkle the spice mixture over it and give it another spin.

Let the cauliflower roast.

Arrange the seasoned cauliflower florets on the baking sheet in a single layer. Roast the cauliflower for 20 to 25 minutes in a preheated oven, tossing halfway through to promote equal cooking, or until it is soft and golden brown.

3. Finally, add little lemon juice: As soon as you take the cauliflower out of the oven, squeeze some fresh lemon juice over it. Toss to mix and add a splash of flavor.

4.Serve and garnish: After roasting, move the cauliflower to a serving platter. Add some freshly cut cilantro as a garnish and, if you'd like, some sesame seeds. Serve hot as a tasty appetizer or as a side dish.

Indian-Spiced Cauliflower is a flavorful recipe that brightens up any dinner with its colorful spices. The mixture of spices has several anti-inflammatory properties in addition to adding rich flavor. This meal is a healthy complement to an anti-inflammatory diet since it's high in fiber, vitamins, and antioxidants.

Recipe 8: Golden Lentil Soup

Servings: 6
Prep Time: 10 minutes
Cook Time: 30 minutes
Total Time: 40 minutes

Ingredients:
-1 tablespoon extra-virgin olive oil
-1 large onion, diced
-3 cloves garlic, minced
-1 tablespoon fresh ginger, minced
-2 medium carrots, diced
-1 teaspoon ground turmeric
-1 teaspoon ground cumin
-1/2 teaspoon ground coriander

- 1/4 teaspoon ground cayenne pepper (optional, for heat)
- 1 cup red lentils, rinsed
- 4 cups low-sodium vegetable broth
- 1 cup coconut milk
- 1 (14-ounce) can diced tomatoes
- 1/2 teaspoon salt
- 1/4 teaspoon black pepper
- 1 cup spinach or kale, chopped
- 1 tablespoon lemon juice (optional)
- Fresh cilantro, chopped (for garnish)

Nutritional Facts (Per Serving):
Calories: 210
Protein: 9g
Carbohydrates: 28g
Dietary Fiber: 9g
Total Sugars: 5g
Total Fat: 8g
Saturated Fat: 5g

Preparation

1. Cook the Fragrances: In a big saucepan, warm the olive oil over medium heat. Saute the chopped onion for four to five

minutes, or until it becomes tender. When aromatic, add the minced garlic and ginger and sauté for an additional minute. Stir in the spices and carrots.

Cook the chopped carrots in the saucepan for three minutes. Add the ground turmeric, coriander, cumin, and, if desired, cayenne pepper and stir. Simmer for an additional one to two minutes to give the spices time to release their scent.

2.Add the tomatoes, broth, and lentils: Add the chopped tomatoes (with their juices), vegetable broth, and red lentils. After bringing the mixture to a boil, turn down the heat. After 20 minutes, or until the carrots and lentils are soft, cover and simmer.

3.Add the greens and coconut milk: Add the chopped spinach or kale, coconut milk, salt, and black pepper and stir. After 5 more minutes of simmering, the greens should be soft and wilted.

4.Finally, add little lemon juice: To enliven the flavors, toss in the lemon juice, if using. If necessary, taste and add additional salt or pepper to suit the seasoning.

5.Serve: Spoon soup into dishes; sprinkle with cilantro that has just been cut. Warm up and serve with naan or crispy bread on the side.

A filling, nourishing, and anti-inflammatory meal, golden lentil soup is infused with warming spices like coriander, cumin, and turmeric. This soup is a hearty and nutritious choice because of the earthy taste of the lentils and the creamy texture of the coconut milk. The soup is ideal for a balanced and anti-inflammatory diet since it is high in protein, fiber, and vital elements.

Recipe 9: Classic Vegetable Broth

Servings: 8 (about 1 cup per serving)
Prep Time: 10 minutes
Cook Time: 1 hour
Total Time: 1 hour 10 minutes

Ingredients:
-2 tablespoons extra-virgin olive oil
-2 large onions, roughly chopped
-3 medium carrots, roughly chopped
-3 celery stalks, roughly chopped
-1 bulb of garlic, halved crosswise
-1 large leek, washed and roughly chopped (white and light green parts only)
-2 medium tomatoes, quartered
-1 small bunch fresh parsley
-2 bay leaves

- 1 teaspoon black peppercorns
- 1 teaspoon dried thyme
- 1 teaspoon salt (or to taste)
- 10 cups water

Nutritional Facts (Per Serving):
Calories: 40
Protein: 1g
Carbohydrates: 7g
Dietary Fiber: 2g
Total Sugars: 3g
Total Fat: 2g

Preparation

1. Get the veggies ready: Chop the celery, onions, carrots, and leek roughly. Quarter the tomatoes and cut the garlic bulb in half crosswise. The veggies will be strained out later, so there's no need to peel them now.
2. Cook the Veggies: Heat the olive oil in a large stockpot over medium heat. Stir in the chopped leek, carrots, celery, and onions. The veggies should be sautéed for 5 to 7 minutes, stirring often, or until they start to soften and take on some color.

3. Add the tomatoes and garlic: Add the quartered tomatoes and the half garlic bulb to the saucepan. Simmer for a further 3–4 minutes, or until the tomatoes begin to soften.

4. Add the water, spices, and herbs: Incorporate the salt, dried thyme, black peppercorns, bay leaves, and fresh parsley. Ten glasses of water should be added. Over medium-high heat, stir to blend well and bring to a boil.

5. Reduce the heat in the broth: Turn down the heat once the soup comes to a boil. Simmer the mixture for 45 to 1 hour with a slightly covered saucepan. The flavors will become more complex the longer you simmer.

Pour the Broth Through Straining

Once the saucepan has reached a simmer, turn off the heat. Pour the broth into a big bowl or another saucepan after carefully straining it through cheesecloth or a fine-mesh sieve, removing the solids. To extract as much liquid as possible, you may use a spoon to push down on the veggies.

6. Modify the seasoning and the storage: If necessary, add extra salt to the seasoning after tasting the soup. The soup should cool fully before being transferred to sealed jars. You may freeze the broth for up to three months or keep it in the fridge for up to five days.

A basic and adaptable recipe for a variety of foods, including soups, stews, and sauces, is classic vegetable broth. Packed with vitamins and minerals, this nutrient-dense soup serves as a nutritious foundation for an anti-inflammatory diet. It's a great way to use up extra veggies and include some natural flavor into different dishes without having to use store-bought broths.

Recipe 10: Stuffed Sweet Potatoes

Servings: 4
Prep Time: 10 minutes
Cook Time: 50 minutes
Total Time: 1 hour

Ingredients:
-4 medium sweet potatoes, scrubbed and pierced with a fork
-1 tablespoon extra-virgin olive oil
-1 small red onion, diced
-2 cloves garlic, minced
-1 red bell pepper, diced
-1 (15-ounce) can black beans, drained and rinsed
-1 teaspoon ground cumin
-1 teaspoon smoked paprika
-1/2 teaspoon ground coriander
-1/2 teaspoon salt

- 1/4 teaspoon black pepper
- 1 cup corn kernels (fresh, frozen, or canned)
- 1/2 cup cherry tomatoes, halved
- 1/4 cup fresh cilantro, chopped
- 1/2 cup shredded cheddar cheese or vegan cheese (optional)
- 1 avocado, diced (for topping)
- 2 tablespoons Greek yogurt or dairy-free yogurt (optional, for topping)
- Lime wedges (for serving)

Nutritional Facts (Per Serving):
Calories: 290
Protein: 7g
Carbohydrates: 53g
Dietary Fiber: 11g
Total Sugars: 10g
Total Fat: 7g
Saturated Fat: 1.5g

Preparation
Sweet potatoes should be baked.
1. Set oven temperature to 400°F, or 200°C. Use parchment paper to line a baking sheet. After piercing the sweet potatoes with a fork, place them on the prepared baking sheet and bake for 40 to 50 minutes, or until they are soft. Depending on the size of the sweet potatoes, cooking times may vary.

2.Get the Filling Ready: In a large pan over medium heat, warm the olive oil while the sweet potatoes are roasting. When the red onion is tender, add it and sauté it for three to four minutes. Once aromatic, add the minced garlic and simmer for an additional minute.

3.Add the spices and vegetables: Cook the chopped red bell pepper in the pan for three to four minutes, or until it starts to soften. Add the ground cumin, coriander, smoked paprika, black beans, salt, and black pepper and stir. Allow the flavors to combine by cooking for two to three minutes.

4.Add the tomatoes and corn: Add the cherry tomatoes and corn kernels, and simmer for a further two minutes, or until the tomatoes are slightly softened and the corn is well cooked. After taking the pan off of the burner, add the chopped cilantro and mix.

5.Incorporate the Sweet Potatoes: After baking, take the sweet potatoes out of the oven and allow them to cool somewhat. Each potato should be cut lengthwise through the middle, then the ends should be gently pressed open. Fluff the sweet potato's inside with a fork.

6. Complete and garnish: Fill the middle of each sweet potato with a spoonful of the prepared black bean and veggie mixture. If preferred, top with vegan or cheddar cheese shreds, then pop back into the oven for five minutes to melt the cheese.

7. Serve: Add some chopped avocado, a dollop of dairy-free or Greek yogurt, and lime wedges on the side to garnish. Savor it hot!

A tasty and high-nutrient choice that is high in fiber, protein, and vitamins are stuffed sweet potatoes. This adaptable recipe, which offers a tasty blend of beans, veggies, and spices to please your palate while nourishing your body, is ideal for a nutritious, anti-inflammatory diet.

Review

Greetings, Reader

We are appreciative that you have selected " The Anti -Inflammatory diet slow cooker cookbook." I sincerely hope that this book has been an invaluable tool for you as you follow the carnivorous diet to a healthier way of living.

I value your opinion much since it enables me to make improvements and provide even better content in the future. I would be very grateful if you could take a few minutes to write a review if you liked this book or found it useful. Not only does your review aid in the discovery of the book by other readers, but it also offers insightful commentary that informs subsequent editions.Would you kindly consider posting your opinions on [enter the name of the website where your book is available for purchase, Amazon.Your input, no matter how brief or in-depth, is greatly appreciated.

Once again, I appreciate your support and wish you great success on your path to fitness and health.

Warm regards ,

Gina P. Erin

Printed in Great Britain
by Amazon